30 Days

To Stop

Overeating

A Mindfulness Program with a Touch of Humor

Harper Daniels

Share your journey!

Let people know you're practicing mindfulness! Post a picture of the cover and include #30DaysNow via social media. Our various guides share the same lessons, so you can see how others are using mindfulness on their journey!

Don't forget that each exercise has a unique hashtag for online sharing.

This book is meant to be a guide only, and does not guarantee specific results. If the lessons and exercises in this book are followed, change can occur for certain people. Results vary from person to person; some people may not need to complete the thirty days to experience change, but it's encouraged that the entire program be read completely through at least once.

The last half of the book consists of blank note pages that the reader can use in conjunction with the exercises for each day. The reader is encouraged to utilize the note pages; though it's not necessary.

Give the gift of mindfulness. See similar guides at www.30DaysNow.com if you wish to purchase a book for a loved one. **See the disclosure below.**

Disclosure (Shared Lessons and Exercises):
Keep in mind that our mindfulness guides share the same lessons and exercises, so there is no need to purchase more than one book; unless you are sharing with a group or giving the guides as gifts. Our mindfulness guides are created for various topics; however, they utilize the same lessons and exercises, so please be aware of this before purchasing. For example, *30 Days to Stop Overeating* will mostly have the same lessons and exercises as *30 Days to Overcome Guilt* and so forth. By reading just one of our guides, you'll be able to apply the same lessons and exercises to multiple areas of your life.

Enjoy your journey of self-discovery!

Contents

Preface

Overeating occurs for various reasons, and it's not necessarily a pernicious habit. However, if you regularly overeat and it's impeding your health, then overeating is a dependency that must be dropped. If you haven't attempted to stop overeating before, it can be a monumental challenge. This 30 day mindfulness program will guide you over the mountain.

For the purpose of this book let's define *overeating* as: an unhealthy dependency on food in the present moment. That may be too broad of a definition, so let's define *unhealthy* as: any amount of food that goes well beyond what's necessary for survival and sustenance. You can define overeating any way you wish – as long as you recognize the habit as a dependency that is supported by adverse thought patterns, feelings, and behaviors.

Of course overeating involves food; that is, we're not talking about the overeating of clothes or bricks. But overeating has little to do with food in general; otherwise we'd all be overeating broccoli, kale, beans, fish, and other healthy foods. This particular dependency involves a complicated reliance on feelings that result from too much intake of specific foods – specifically those foods high in sugar, sodium, and fat, as those trigger certain brain chemicals and reactions that we become conditioned to rely on. In time, the dependency strengthens and takes more of a foothold. This negative reliance is common in modern society, since high sugar, high sodium, and high fat foods are household staples. So, if you have an overeating problem, don't be ashamed - you're not alone. This program will help you drop the dependency.

The following pages involve a 30 day program made up of lessons and exercises to help you overcome thought patterns, feelings, and behaviors that have you regularly overeating. Though these lessons and exercises can be applied to any adverse reliance, this program will focus specifically on the problem of overeating.

For some readers, they'll overcome quickly and will drop the unhealthy thoughts and habits in no time; and for others, they'll overcome gradually. In either case, if you stick with the program, you'll start to witness your dependency weaken. Don't critique your progress, as this isn't a competition and there isn't a goal you must attain. Let the debilitating thoughts, feelings, and dependency simply drop as you work through the exercises and lessons.

It's not necessary to complete these days in order, nor should you be religious about completing them successfully. There is no such thing as a successful completion of this program. The bottom line is to observe and awaken, and that cannot be obtained through success, force, pressure, struggle, or competition. Simply relax, follow the program, and the grip of overeating will loosen.

You'll also notice that mindfulness, silence, and stillness are a regular discipline for each day. Because you've been influenced by a dependency based society that demands instant gratification, silence and stillness may seem nearly impossible for you to practice. For this reason, we'll incorporate this discipline from the outset. A quiet and still mind is an incredibly powerful resource, but one that requires daily maintenance.

It should also be noted that you're not required to quit overeating during this program. The point being: by practicing the following exercises and lessons in the days to come, you won't even need willpower to stop – it'll just happen.

One of the most important lessons to keep in mind is to not fight the constraint while participating in this program. Dependencies, habits, and strong patterns of thinking are empowered by a fight and struggle. Keep overeating for the length of this program without regret or remorse; unless you witness it drop – then let it go. Overeating, like most unhealthy habits, feeds on negative thought patterns, fear, and struggle. This program will help you overcome without a conflict.

You'll need about 15-30 minutes per day for the program; but feel free to spend more time if needed. The amount of time doesn't matter, as long as you're in an environment that allows you to concentrate without distraction. Also to be mentioned, the last portion of this book includes note pages that you can use with the exercises. It's encouraged that you write down any thoughts, insights, adaptations, lessons, mantras, etc...on those blank pages. The note pages can also be used to rip out and take with you. Feel free to use them as you wish.

One last thing: If you're like most people, you might dependent on caffeine or alcohol to some extent. If you are, do your best to lessen the consumption of these substances over the next 30 days. Can you cut consumption of these substances in half, or more? It's important that your mind is sober and your body relaxed to make the most of these exercises.

Let's get started.

Let others know you're practicing mindfulness! Post a picture of the cover and include #30DaysNow. Also, don't forget that each exercise has a unique hashtag for online sharing.

Day 1

Exercise:

Find a place without distraction, and turn off all electronics. Sit with your back straight, kneel, or lie on a hard surface (not bed) and remain in silence for 10 minutes.

During these 10 minutes, take deep and focused breaths and hold them for a few seconds each. Exhale slowly. Listen intently to your breathing. Don't try to change it – simply listen, and feel the air go in and out.

*When you're ready, repeat the mantra: "**Be still. Be silent.**" Repeat this slowly multiple times out loud as well as quietly. You might experience boredom or anxiety, but continue repeating the mantra regardless. Repeat it until you're calm and focused. You can continue the deep breathing during the mantra, or take deep breaths during pauses. Don't rush.*

Each of the 30 days will have this time of silence, focused breathing, and a mantra. Except for this page, the end of each day will remind you of the minutes you are to spend in silence and focused breathing; and will also have a mantra for you to practice. You can repeat the mantras during your times of silence and focused breathing, or following. Remember, there is no right or wrong way to do this.

Dependencies want to fight; in fact, they're energized by fighting. Instead of fighting the habit of overeating, meet it with silence and observation. Let the exercises and lessons in this program guide you.

Day 2

Exercise:

Ponder this question: Can you remember a time in your life when you didn't overeat on a regular basis?

Writing is extremely beneficial to the mind; especially when pondering. Write down your thoughts about this particular question. If your mind drifts, then write whatever thoughts emerge. It's okay if you have nothing to write, but ponder the question regardless.

Were you able to remember a period in your life when you didn't overeat often? If you're like many people in western civilization, you may have to return to memories of childhood to determine that period. It's not uncommon for a person to learn to overeat at an early age. Someone might start overeating because of family customs or tradition, witnessing a parent use food to cope with stress, or having a friend group that encourages overeating.

Recognize that overeating is a learned behavior with roots. However, it can be dropped quickly and completely; and you have the capability to drop it.

*10 minutes of silence and focused breathing. Repeat the mantra: ***"Drop. Unlearn. Discover."**

Day 3

Exercise:

On a piece of paper (any size) write down the goals that you've been striving to achieve – i.e. the goals that you believe will bring you fulfillment. For example: a new job, a house in a nice neighborhood, traveling the world, a business, a family, new friends, a degree or certification, building a network, reaching a net worth of a million dollars, etc.

Now, tear up the paper into multiple pieces and throw away.

Goals can be very helpful and useful if they're not obsessed over. However, in the modern world people develop a reliance on goals. Think about all the times you've said something like, *"I need to get that," "I must reach this," "I'll do anything to accomplish that"*, etc. It's often the case that people spend more time worrying about their goals, than freely doing something in the present moment to reach them. Plus, the goal in itself is fleeting, while the journey in the present moment is real and lasting.

The habit of thinking that goals must be met, or else failure ensues, is subtly fixed to dependencies. When you've overeaten in the past, what was the goal? What was it that you felt you needed to achieve?

*10 minutes of silence and focused breathing. Repeat the mantra: *"My happiness does not depend on meeting a goal. I'm happy now."*

Day 4

Exercise:

Stand still for 5 minutes; with knees slightly bent (i.e. your legs should not be locked). At first try to remain still, but then let your body sway. Let it move any way it wishes. Feel its movement. If you're unable to stand, you can do this same exercise by extending your arm or leg from a sitting position – try to keep it straight, but then let go of trying and allow movement to happen.

We tend to lock ourselves into particular goals, expectations, thought patterns, and habits. We even go so far as to admire and honor rigidity – people mistake rigidity for perseverance. This is taught and told to us by our culture. Everything around you may be shouting, even in a quiet whisper, that you must remain submissive and obedient.

Overeating, like most dependencies, is no different in its message. It wants you to remain rigid; not to be released from its hold. If you freely moved on from overeating, it would lose you as a dependent. By the way, who wants to remain rigidly dependent on something like overeating food for their happiness? Or I should say…false happiness.

The message of overeating essentially says, *"You need to eat as much food as possible to feel satisfied and happy."* Allow your body and mind to move on from overeating. Trust that your body and mind will sway to its own rhythm, and away from the desire to overeat.

*10 minutes of silence and focused breathing. Repeat the mantra: *"**I am now free to move. I am free to move on.**"*

Day 5

Exercise:

Taste something by eating it very slowly for at least 5 minutes. Pick something with a lot of flavor: a piece of fruit, a strong tea, a spice, soup with many ingredients, honey, etc. Close your eyes through most of your tasting. Savor the piece of food slowly. Pay close attention to the feel of the taste on your tongue. Chew slowly.

Overeating does a great job at stealing presence away from the other senses, as do many dependencies. Since overeating is directly related satiation, the more those senses are abused the more our other senses are neglected. When was the last time you thoroughly enjoyed the taste of an orange, vanilla, dark chocolate, olive oil, or cheese? I don't mean enjoying the flavor for a few seconds and then continuing on to eat, but to let the flavor linger before taking another bite.

The taste of a pineapple, pepper, grape, or apple is far more real and satisfying than filling the stomach to max capacity. It may sound silly to say that, but it's true, because those tastes are based in reality. You can actually interact with them in the present, and they don't hypnotize you into an illusory relationship like overeating does.

Let the taste of food bring you into the present moment. Overeating doesn't allow you to thoroughly enjoy taste. Taste the present, and let the habit of overeating drop.

*10 minutes of silence and focused breathing. Repeat the mantra: *"I am free to taste."*

Day 6

Exercise:

On a sheet of paper (any size) write down all the internal lies that you regularly hear about yourself – i.e. within your mind.

Now, tear the paper into multiple pieces, and throw away.

It's common to have an internal voice (or voices) within your mind, playing a record of lies over and over. We eventually begin to accept these lies and let them impact our growth and happiness. Most people you see on a daily basis have these recurring internal voices; and most people are oblivious to them – sort of like white noise. This isn't a mental illness, but a way in which the mind works. We all experience these internal quiet voices whispering untruths about our being. These lies are nothing to fear, but they need to be observed. Writing them down can help you observe and become aware of their deceptions.

The power of silence, focused breathing, and mantras, which you have been practicing, is to draw out the lies. Let them manifest, and observe them. Common internal lies include: *"You are a loser," "You have become nothing, and you will never improve," "You are worthless. No one likes you," "You'll always be alone," "You're a burden,"* and so on. These thoughts are not part of you; however, the deception is to make you believe they are. Like many common habits in our culture, overeating implants many of these lies clandestinely.

*10 minutes of silence and focused breathing. Repeat the mantra: **"Thoughts are only thoughts - nothing more."**

Day 7

Exercise:

For 10 minutes, look at your face in a mirror. Analyze its curvature, look closely at the color of your eyes, notice the blemishes and spots, observe its movements, etc. Look at your face as if you were observing someone else's. Do this without judgment, but observe any thoughts that emerge.

Did you experience judgment? Were you upset? Was this an uncomfortable exercise? Were you content with the look of your face? Did any thoughts appear?

Rarely do we stop to look at our faces in a mirror for an extended period of time. You may for a quick moment while cleaning or dressing, but hardly long enough to see its uniqueness. The face may be the most important part of your body, since it's what people recognize most. However, the face that you have is not "you."

Judgment runs rampant today. Even those who say, *"I don't judge. I never judge a person"* are fooling themselves. It takes a lot of practice and mindfulness to be judgment free. It's possible to reach that awareness, but it needs to start with your perception of "you." The day you stop judging yourself, including your appearance, you'll stop judging others.

The hope of overeating is that you will diligently judge yourself, consciously and subconsciously, so that you'll seek validation within the confines of its illusion.

*10 minutes of silence and focused breathing. Repeat the mantra: **"I am not my face. I do not need validation."**

Day 8

Exercise:

Say the words "Guilt", "Shame", and "Regret" 10 times to yourself out loud. Don't rush. Pause between each repetition. For the pause, you can take a deep breath. Your eyes can remain open or closed. Again, don't rush - say the words slowly and observe any thoughts, feelings, or images that emerge internally.

Now, say these words again 10 times, but with a smile.

What futile credence we give words such as Guilt, Shame and Regret. We use these words on ourselves as well as others; they become regular vocabulary for our internal recurring voices. And in the end, they're mere words that hold no power. What would these words be without a facial expression, tone, inflection, or emphasis?

When you said these three specific words, what thoughts came to mind, what did you feel, and was there a reaction in your body? If there is a reaction, such as shortness of breath or a frown, people tend to interpret it as sadness; but this reaction is a learned behavior. We've been taught to feel and think a certain way with regard to guilt, shame, and regret. The truth is: these words mean nothing.

The habit of overeating, like most dependencies, flourishes on these three words and the learned reactions they produce. But see them for what they are...mere words with no power.

*10 minutes of silence and focused breathing. Repeat the mantra: *__*"I am not Guilt, Shame, or Regret."*__

Day 9

Exercise:

Deliberately feel the sensation of water on your skin for at least 5 minutes. You can do this exercise in the shower, while washing your hands, taking a bath, going for a swim, walking in the rain, or simply placing your hand in a sink filled with water. Close your eyes if you like.

How often do you deliberately experience the essence of water? We take it for granted every day. It's a remarkable chemical substance in the universe that is necessary for all life. Without it, we wouldn't exist. This one transparent and fluid substance has immense capacity. A large percentage of your physical body is made of this natural substance. Experience it.

Every day we jump in the shower, wash our hands, and drink it – but rarely do we take time to slowly and deliberately appreciate our natural response to water. Overeating can never give you the joy, energy, sensation, reality, and present moment that water can give. Water is an example of a positive dependency that doesn't bind you emotionally or spiritually. Water doesn't need you; the habit of overeating, however, does.

There are many lessons that water can teach: fluidity, flow, evaporation, change, motion, stillness, and life. You can't get any of those lessons through a dependency such as overeating; or any unnatural dependency for that matter.

*10 minutes of silence and focused breathing. Repeat the mantra: *"I am fluid. I change. I flow."*

Day 10

Exercise:

Count to 25 slowly, pausing for a few seconds before the next number; then, count backward from 25 slowly. Try this with your eyes closed. While counting up you can imagine yourself being lifted into the sky; and then while counting down, descending back to earth.

Our world today is about speed. Everyone seems to be in a rush, yet most of people are unsatisfied; and, they have no clue where they're going. Chasing the next best thing is a fruitless endeavor. It's the rare person who slows down to enjoy the present moment, regardless of its nature. Because there seems to be so many problems, and most jobs are focused on resolving those problems, people are compelled to accept anxiety and rush toward a reward and conclusion. That surely isn't happiness. Happiness can only be found in the present moment, not in a hypothetical future of rewards and successes. Rushing is another form of going nowhere.

How many times have you rushed through a meal? This is destructive to your peace of mind and health: concentration suffers, stress levels rise, and awareness to the present moment isn't possible. Try this exercise while overeating.

It's critical to slow down. You only have one life to live – don't rush through it, and don't be dependent on anything that encourages you to rush. Be still, and slow down.

*10 minutes of silence and focused breathing. Repeat the mantra: *"Slow down. Do not rush. Enjoy the present moment."*

Day 11

(Share this experience using #30DaysDoorway)

Exercise:

Stand in front of a doorway, with the door open. Close your eyes, and take a deep breath. With eyes closed and holding your breath, step through the doorway. Once you have stepped through completely, open your eyes and exhale.

Doorways are amazing tools that can be used for practicing mindfulness and observation. How often do you rush through doors without paying attention to the change of environment? We don't often pay attention or appreciate the transition; we simply rush through unaware that our perspective has changed. This isn't a bad thing; in fact, it's great that we don't stall in front of doorways, too afraid to enter the next environment. At the beginning of this exercise you were in a particular place, and then you stepped through a doorway into a completely different setting. You made a transition without worry or concern, and very naturally.

When it comes to physical doorways, we rarely stop and worry about the change of environment – we just walk through and accept the new experience. You can apply this same lesson to decisions that have you stressed, anxious, or worried. Naturally step through the decision to drop your dependency on overeating, and accept the change; but try to step through aware and grateful.

*10 minutes of silence and focused breathing. Repeat the mantra: ***"I accept change with awareness and gratitude."***

Day 12

Exercise:

Observe your body. Observe how it feels, moves, and reacts. More direction is explained below.

If you're still overeating, observe your body movements, sounds, sensations, and breaths during the overeating experience. Do your eyes look down or roll? Do you move your hands fast or slow? Is there a stopping and starting at certain intervals? Are you making certain noises? How is your posture? Try to observe everything about your body while overeating. Be aware of its affect on your body.

If you are not overeating today, then continue with the 10 minutes of silence and focused breathing, but get in touch with your body. A good way to do this is by touching each body part and saying its name, leaving your hand on the part for a few seconds and feeling its texture and warmth. Start with your head: place your hand on your head and say, *"I am touching my head."* And then work your way down to your shoulders, arms, stomach, legs, knees, and feet. Focus your attention on one body part at a time. Say its name and describe what you are touching.

*10 minutes of silence and focused breathing. Repeat the mantra: **"I am not my body."***

Day 13
(Share this experience using #30DaysPassing)

Exercise:

On a piece of paper (any size) write down the name of your current emotion. For example, at this moment you might be feeling agitated, calm, bored, angry, anxious, excited, etc. Whatever emotion you are experiencing, give it a name and put it on paper.

Now, write down "I'm experiencing this emotion in the present moment and it will pass. It's only an emotion."

You can throw the paper away, or hold onto it if you wish.

Similar to how we give certain words credence, we tend to give our emotions a lot of trust. We also tend to blame the outside world for emotions we are feeling: *"They made me angry," "I'm depressed because they didn't want me," "If they gave me the job, I would be happy."*

The emotions you feel are in you, not in the outer world. No one can cause you to feel or emote in a particular way; if they're able to, it's only because you let them. A great way to let a harmful emotion pass is to observe it; and a good start is by giving it a name and seeing it as powerless.

It's commonplace to blame others for our pain. Instead of seeing the emotion for what it is and letting it pass, we've been taught to rely on dependencies, like overeating, to manage the emotional reaction. Wake up! Emotions are not you.

*10 minutes of silence and focused breathing. Repeat the mantra: **"I am not an emotion. All emotions pass."**

Day 14

Exercise:

This exercise may seem frivolous, but give it a try; because it may be one of the lessons that benefit you most.

For the remainder of the day, whenever you use the bathroom, for any reason, take your time with what you're doing. Don't rush through the process, like you may normally do. Focus on taking your time in the bathroom; do every step of your bathroom experience twice as slow. It may even help to say each step: "I am now sitting up straight on the toilet," "I am now putting soap on my hands," "I am now drying my hands," etc.

Most people hurry up their bathroom experience, not realizing what they're doing – forcing, not standing or sitting straight, not relaxing, not washing their hands properly, not drying their hands slowly. They rush in and out, like they have somewhere important to go. Don't be like that any longer. Take your time in the bathroom; it's not only unhealthy for the body to rush the excretion process, but it's also unhealthy for the mind. A rushed bathroom experience doesn't allow you to live in the present moment. Allow the excretion and cleaning to happen naturally with relaxed and focused attention.

By practicing this exercise, you'll build the discipline to slow down; and this is an incredibly powerful discipline to apply when eating food. Overeating wants you to rush; so slow down considerably. .

*10 minutes of silence and focused breathing. Repeat the mantra: **"Don't hurry. Stay present. Stay still."**

Day 15

Exercise:

Light a candle and observe its flame for 5 minutes. Watch it move and feel its heat. Appreciate its energy.

Now, blow out the flame.

(If you don't have a candle, light a match and blow it out; and if you don't have a candle or match, stare at a dim light for 5 minutes and then turn it off.)

The temperature of a small candle flame (and match flame) is around 1200 Celsius (which is about 2000 Fahrenheit). That's a lot of energy! And within a fraction of a second, it was extinguished as you blew it out; or in the case of the light, turned off its energy source. There wasn't a gradual process with delays and stops. You blew out the highly energized flame, and that was it - from 1200 Celsius to nonexistent in no time; or should I say, in present no time.

We think that our dependencies have so much energy and power. It's not just the habit of overeating, but all dependencies survive on this deception of power. The truth is that dependencies don't have energy like the candle flame, though your mind may have been tricked into believing they do. The candle flame is real and powerful; whereas dependencies are illusory and fictitious.

As easily and quickly as you extinguished the flame, you can drop a dependency in the present moment.

*10 minutes of silence and focused breathing. Repeat the mantra: **"Dependency isn't real. It can be extinguished."**

(21)

Day 16

Exercise:

Today, look for the color blue in your surrounding environment. If possible, spend the entire day looking for the color blue in the places you go. Whether you're doing this exercise in a bedroom, office, classroom, outside, or while traveling, look for the color blue in all things that surround you. If you think you'll forget to do this throughout the entire day, spend at least 20 focused minutes practicing this exercise at some point.

Focused attention is something that must be practiced - it doesn't come easy in our rapid paced society. Instead of encouraging us to focus and observe, the modern world encourages us to rush and get things done.

Searching for a color or shape helps to slow down our accelerated and cyclical thought patterns, and reminds us that there's more to the world than the chaotic thoughts we collectively and daily experience. By searching for the color blue, your mind can escape the fictitious grip of anxiety, lust, desire, depression, worry, fear, or any other potent emotion. When you are overeating, are you aware of the colors around you? Most likely not.

The habit of overeating functions to distract your conscience from present reality. Look for the color blue today, and wake up to life in the present moment.

*15 minutes of silence and focused breathing. Repeat the mantra: *"I am focused, here and now."*

Day 17

Exercise:

Go out and buy a small trash can. You should be able to find one cheaply. If you don't have the funds for this exercise, you can use an empty box or container; however, a small trash can works better for its symbolism.

Designate this specific trash can your "concerns and worries can" (or use any title you wish) – some people benefit from writing this label directly onto the can.

Now, write down (on scraps of paper or whatever paper you wish to use) any concerns, worries, and adverse thoughts that you may be experiencing today, and throw them into the can. Try to practice this every day: quickly write down worries, concerns, and negative thoughts, and then throw them into the can. It may be beneficial to have a supply of scrap paper near the can for easy access.

This exercise may seem simple, but let's go beyond throwing your written concerns, worries, and thoughts away. Designate a few times during the week for sifting through the can and taking out random worries and concerns from days prior – just reach in and pull some out. Observe them, but don't judge yourself. This is a great exercise to learn your negative thought patterns and the lies that grip your conscience. If you stick with this practice, you may gain a deeper understanding into the dependencies, habits, thought patterns, and feelings that accompany overeating.

*15 minutes of silence and focused breathing. Repeat the mantra: **"There is nothing to worry about. All is well."**

Day 18

Exercise:

Write a letter or email to yourself. There is something about using pen and paper that is very effective when writing letters, but feel free to write an email if you wish. Don't send the letter or email, just write it and save it for a day – you can toss it out or delete it tomorrow.

Write anything that comes to mind: It can be advice you want to give yourself, a story from the past, random thoughts and feelings, frustrations and worries, things you're thankful for, etc. There is no right or wrong – write whatever comes to mind in the moment. Try to write at least two full paragraphs.

What was the theme and voice of your message? Was it a positive or negative tone? Were you advising yourself? Did you make any judgments about yourself? Did you start demanding that you should or should not do something? Was the letter full of gratitude? Was there anger and despair? Read the letter as if you were reading it from a friend – is it a letter that would upset you, or one that you would welcome with excitement and a smile?

Whatever you wrote is essentially being written on the tablet of your mind. This exercise is useful for getting to know the internal voice that we all have in our minds. It's an internal voice that can change for the better with observation, acceptance, and awareness. Be aware of your internal voice in the present moment.

*15 minutes of silence and focused breathing. Repeat the mantra: "**I am not my internal voice. I am aware.**"

Day 19

Exercise:

Find a hard object that you can hold in the palm of your hand (such as a stone, ball, or bottle). With either hand, grip this object tightly and squeeze it as hard as you can. Squeeze it forcefully until you can't hold on to it any longer. Drop the object when ready.

If you could continue squeezing that object forever, perhaps you would; but your muscles and nerves can only endure for so long. At some point, you simply and quickly release the grip and drop the object. There isn't a process to the drop; it just happens when your body says that's enough. The release happens naturally without effort.

Letting go of an unhealthy dependency, habit, thought pattern, addiction, emotion, or behavior can be that easy. Letting go can be as natural and guilt free as dropping the object you were gripping on to so tightly in this exercise; so, take a lesson from your body's experience. When it's time to let go, then let go. The time to let go is always now. Just let the drop happen.

The time to stop overeating is always…now.

*15 minutes of silence and focused breathing. Repeat the mantra: **"Letting go is natural. I can let go, here and now."**

Day 20

Exercise:

Choose a physical symbol that will remind you to observe and be aware in the present moment. Try to choose something from nature, or that is made of natural material.

The object you choose can be anything, but it's best if it's something that you can enjoy looking at and touching. For example, many walkers and hikers will find a unique rock small enough to carry in their hands. A stone, necklace, bracelet, seashell, cedar block, coin...anything will do, as long as you enjoy it and you can dedicate it as a tool for remembrance.

Another cunning trick of the overeating habit is to confuse the mind into forgetting you're part of the natural world. By having a symbol of remembrance, you can reconnect with the present moment and the essence of creation. This symbol isn't meant to be an idol, god, or icon. Don't think too deeply into this. The symbol is simply a tool to help you remember where you are in the here and now. As long as you're aware of the present, you'll have no desire to return to the habit of overeating.

*15 minutes of silence and focused breathing. Repeat the mantra: "**All is well. Here and now, all is well.**"

Day 21

Exercise:

Look at a picture or painting for 10 minutes, alone, in silence, and without any distraction. It would be best if the picture isn't of family or friends, but it could have been created by someone you know. Try to choose a work of art for this exercise, but any picture or painting will suffice.

When the thought of excess food occupies the mind, there's a loss of connection to images that can be helpful to the awakened mind. The purpose of this exercise is to return the mind to an appreciation of truly inventive and innovative art. A printed picture hanging in a cheap motel room has more artistry than the largest chocolate bar, case of beer, pizza, or burrito.

Observing a picture, photo, or print for an extended period of time can aid the mind in slowing down. You may have had a photo of a landscape hanging in your home for many years, but have you ever taken the time to carefully analyze it? Take some time and do that. Appreciate the image, and observe your thoughts in the process.

*15 minutes of silence and focused breathing. Repeat the mantra: **"Stillness. Silence. Peace. Presence."**

Day 22

Exercise:

Go for a mindfulness walk for at least 10 minutes. Focus on each step. Feel the steps: the feel of your feet hitting the ground, your heel rolling forward, your toes, the bend of your knees, your hips working to balance your posture, the swinging of your arms, etc. Don't rush; go slow. Focus on your breathing as well. Get in tune with your body. Pay attention to your physical senses throughout the walk. Focus – don't listen to music or be distracted.

Human beings have always used walking as a naturally restorative exercise. There is something about walking, and focusing on the walk, that calms the mind and soul. The longer one walks, the more relaxed one feels.

Any moment is a good time to walk and experience your inner and outer environment. During long walks, thoughts will emerge that will allow you to consciously observe them. Let the thoughts pass; you may even have emotions that emerge, observe those and let them pass as well. Focusing on your steps will help you clear the mind of clutter. Walking in the early morning and at dusk is especially beneficial.

A 20 minute walk brings more comfort, stillness, peace, focus, and awareness than overeating a thousand times. Walk every day, as much as you can.

*15 minutes of silence and focused breathing. Repeat the mantra: *"I am relaxed. I am at peace."*

Day 23

Exercise:

Hold a smile for 5 minutes. You don't need to do this exercise in front of a mirror; but feel free to do so if you wish. You can even do this exercise during the 15 minutes of silence and focused breathing. While holding your smile, take a moment and feel your face; actually touch the smile and the curvature of your lips and cheek bones.

Have you ever behaved a certain way and then saw your mood change immediately? Physical exercise, such as running and weightlifting, does this for many people. Certain forms of yoga have also been used by people to change their moods. The point is: changing your behavior not only impacts other people, but can also impact your perception of yourself.

You'll notice that while you're smiling during this exercise, you may experience certain emotions. You might feel silly, embarrassed, stupid, funny, weird, or whatever. Continue smiling regardless. In fact, if you are still overeating at this point in the program, smile while you're overeating – hold the smile until you are through eating; set a reminder alarm if needed. As always, observe your thoughts while you're smiling; observe the thoughts as if they're clouds passing by in a bright blue sky.

Smiling causes an authentic reaction in our bodies and minds that is essentially good. The present moment enjoys a nice smile. So hold that smile until you no longer can.

*15 minutes of silence and focused breathing. Repeat the mantra: *"**Happiness is now. I am happy.**"*

Day 24

Exercise:

Spend 5 minutes smelling something aromatic: a piece of fruit, a spice, tea, pine, cedar, a flower, a scented candle, etc. Focus on the smell of that one thing for the entire 5 minutes. Don't let anything distract you from the smell.

How often do you take time to enjoy a fragrant smell? One of the lies of modern society is that if you stop and enjoy your five senses for too long, you'll miss out on…fill in the blank. While people are rushing toward their goals with stress levels spiking, they're totally missing out on awareness in the present moment. People stare at images of food that others have posted on the internet, but don't take the time to smell or taste real food in the present moment.

What's better: overeating, or enjoying the smell of vanilla, orange, or pine in the present moment? The first is harmful and illusory; the second is real and sensational. The habit of overeating does a great job from stealing time and energy from your other senses, such as smell. One of the best ways get into the present moment and away from an illusion is through focusing on smell and the use of your other senses. Don't let overeating diminish your other senses any longer.

*15 minutes of silence and focused breathing. Repeat the mantra: "**I can sense the present.**"

Day 25

Exercise:

Think of a major worry that consistently upsets you. On a sheet of paper, write down three worst case scenarios for that dominating concern. For example, if someone is persistently worried about dying alone, that individual can write as a worst case scenario, "I will die alone, without anyone at my side, and without family or loved ones to say goodbye." As mentioned, write down three worst case scenarios for the worry. The worry doesn't have to be as extreme as dying alone; use whichever worry hinders you.

Now, next to each of those three worst case scenarios write, "I accept this." You can either toss the paper or keep it.

Worry is an illness that goes untreated in most people. Think of worry like a cancer of the spirit; but few people know how to treat it effectively. One of the only ways to eradicate worry isn't to fight, ignore, or run from it; but to face it in the present moment and accept it for the illusion it is. You can never be worried about something happening in the present moment – that's impossible; you can only be worried about the future, which is always illusory.

Writing down your worries and worst case scenarios, if they ever do come true (which they rarely do), is a great way to draw those thoughts out of your mind and into the present moment, allowing you to face, accept, and observe them. Overeating only exacerbates worries and anxieties.

*15 minutes of silence and focused breathing. Repeat the mantra: **"Worries are not real. They are passing thoughts."**

(31)

Day 26

(Share this experience using #30DaysPinch)

Exercise:

Pinch the skin on the back of your hand or forearm until there is discomfort and slight pain. It's not necessary to pinch hard enough to bruise yourself, just enough to feel a small burn.

Did I cause the pain by asking you to do this exercise? No; you caused this pain to yourself – think about this carefully. You even decided how much pain to give yourself, and when to relieve the pain. You can't blame me or anyone else for the pain you just experienced. You were solely responsible. You were also responsible for letting go.

This is easily understood with regard to physical pain, such as pinching oneself; however, we have a lot of difficulty understanding this lesson as it applies to adverse emotions and feelings. How often have you said, and have heard others say, *"He makes me so angry when...", "I'm depressed because she...",* or *"I'm so frustrated that they..."* No person ever makes you experience negative feelings. It's always you who are experiencing them; and then placing the blame on others. Essentially, you are emotionally pinching yourself and not letting go. People go their entire lives without releasing the pinch. Instead of letting go, they scream at others, *"Release the pain! Let go! Fix this! Stop this! You're to blame!"* Wake up and see that you are solely responsible for letting go of the pain, and you can do it now.

*15 minutes of silence and focused breathing. Repeat the mantra: **"I can release negative feelings, here and now."**

Day 27

Exercise:

For 5 minutes, hum to yourself with mouth and eyes closed. Take deep breaths between pauses. You can do this exercise lying on a hard floor, standing, kneeling, or sitting with back straight.

This exercise may seem cliché, but there is a lot that can be learned from the sound of your own voice during a long hum. Humming relaxes the body and mind – similar to listening to rain drops, crickets in the evening, leaves rustling, or a waterfall. It is believed the reason for this relaxing effect involves the wavelengths produced and sent in perpetual flow.

But what's especially interesting about your humming is that it's directly related to your breathing. If you take shorter, rushed breaths, your hum won't be as long and effective; but if you take concentrated, deep breaths, then your hum will serve to relax your body, and possibly bring you into present moment awareness. Also, did you notice that it was you who was relaxing you? You weren't dependent on overeating food to become calm and still.

From time to time, listen to yourself hum; listen to the wavelengths you produce from your own being. This is always available to you in the present moment.

*15 minutes of silence and focused breathing. Repeat the mantra: **"Calmness and stillness are always present."**

Day 28

Exercise:

Find a coin. While standing, flip the coin and let it land wherever. If it lands with the head side up, spin around to the right until you come back to your original place; if it lands tail side up, spin around to the left until you come back to your original place. Again, head side up, spin to the right; tail side up, spin to the left – doing a full circle until you return to your original standing position.

In which direction did you spin? In this exercise you left the direction of your movement completely up to the flip, the coin, and gravity. When you spun, you experienced a specific visual perception of the environment that you would not have had from spinning in the opposite direction. But, you returned to the original position regardless, full circle.

The experience would have been different if you spun to the opposite side; and if you repeat this exercise multiple times, your experiences in the same direction will be different as well. The point being: it doesn't matter what direction you go in or what you experience; you'll always return to the present moment; so the time to be awake, aware, and happy is always now. Overeating will never get you closer to happiness in the present moment; you have it, here and now.

*15 minutes of silence and focused breathing. Repeat the mantra: **"The direction does not matter. I am always here and now, in the present moment."**

Day 29

Exercise:

Make yourself laugh for 5 minutes. Don't stop laughing. You might feel strange, weird, embarrassed, or stupid...it doesn't matter, just laugh. Try to laugh alone and without the aid of a comedy or joke. If you don't know how to start, just start making the noises that typically accompany your laughter.

What feelings did you experience during this exercise? Many people report feeling embarrassed or goofy, which is great; however, most people also report a feeling of relief and buoyancy when they've completed this exercise.

Similar to holding a smile, laughing for 5 minutes is a fantastic way to come into present awareness. If you think about it, humor is necessary for life. How sad is the person who is unable to laugh at the experiences of life? After all, life is funny, even the dreadful and lousy experiences.

If you ever again experience adverse thoughts and feelings that accompany overeating, simply laugh at them. Consider how crazy and frivolous the habit of overeating and your reactions to it are; it really is a funny dependency. No other living thing on the planet becomes dependent on overeating food. The entire situation is comical. If you perceive the habit for what it truly is - a fictitious, impractical, and frivolous dependency – then it can be easily dropped. You must learn to laugh at it. Genuinely laugh the habit away.

*15 minutes of silence and focused breathing. Repeat the mantra: **"Life is wonderful, funny, and real."**

Day 30

Exercise:

Take a piece of paper (one that you can keep) and write down all that you are grateful for – these things don't have to be in any particular order of importance.

Next to each thing you list, write "Thank you."

The person who isn't thankful for all that life gives is typically quite miserable; and the habit of overeating thrives on that misery. The truly grateful person can let go of anything at anytime. A thankful person is always a happy person, so practice gratitude daily.

Have you ever heard anyone say, *"I'm so grateful to overeat"*? Nobody is thankful for overeating; which is a clear sign that it's a destructive dependency. However, a few people who have overeaten have learned to be thankful for the present moment experience.

Not only is it unhealthy, but overeating discourages a grateful mind and soul. With only one life to live in the present moment, it's important to always emphasize a grateful heart. Spend time with people who are grateful, and do things that nourish a thankful heart in the present moment. Anything that encourages misery and depression isn't worth giving attention to. Be thankful, always.

*15 minutes of silence and focused breathing. Repeat the mantra: *"I am grateful. I am thankful."*

Conclusion

The exercises and lessons in this program taught and encouraged observation, awareness to your present moment experience, change of perception, and awakening to true happiness, which can only be found here and now. You were shown that your negative thoughts and feelings are not caused by overeating, or any unhealthy reliance, but are solely within you and illusory; which means that you are capable of letting those thoughts and feelings pass and dropping your dependency on overeating.

As mentioned at the beginning, there were no goals or measures of success for this program. If you were hoping to find a reason to eat less or eat more, then you may be spending too much time struggling and thinking about overeating. This was not meant to be a struggle, but a release.

Life is not meant to be spent overeating, or relying on any toxic dependency. Wake up to the present moment and enjoy your present experience. If you've made it through the program, you are certainly more awakened than when you started; however, don't give up mindfully practicing observation of thoughts and feelings, stillness, silence, deep and focused breathing, allowing everything to pass, laughing, smiling, and being grateful.

Live wonderfully awakened and aware...overeating or otherwise.

Notes for Day 1

(Use this page to write down thoughts, reminders, ideas, prayers, mantras, revelations, lessons, modifications to the exercise, or experiences. If you'd like to share something, please post using **#30DaysNow** or use the exercise's unique hashtag.)

Notes for Day 2

(Use this page to write down thoughts, reminders, ideas, prayers, mantras, revelations, lessons, modifications to the exercise, or experiences. If you'd like to share something, please post using **#30DaysNow** or use the exercise's unique hashtag.)

Notes for Day 3

(Use this page to write down thoughts, reminders, ideas, prayers, mantras, revelations, lessons, modifications to the exercise, or experiences. If you'd like to share something, please post using **#30DaysNow** or use the exercise's unique hashtag.)

Notes for Day 4

(Use this page to write down thoughts, reminders, ideas, prayers, mantras, revelations, lessons, modifications to the exercise, or experiences. If you'd like to share something, please post using **#30DaysNow** or use the exercise's unique hashtag.)

Notes for Day 5

(Use this page to write down thoughts, reminders, ideas, prayers, mantras, revelations, lessons, modifications to the exercise, or experiences. If you'd like to share something, please post using **#30DaysNow** or use the exercise's unique hashtag.)

Notes for Day 6

(Use this page to write down thoughts, reminders, ideas, prayers, mantras, revelations, lessons, modifications to the exercise, or experiences. If you'd like to share something, please post using **#30DaysNow** or use the exercise's unique hashtag.)

Notes for Day 7

(Use this page to write down thoughts, reminders, ideas, prayers, mantras, revelations, lessons, modifications to the exercise, or experiences. If you'd like to share something, please post using **#30DaysNow** or use the exercise's unique hashtag.)

Notes for Day 8

(Use this page to write down thoughts, reminders, ideas, prayers, mantras, revelations, lessons, modifications to the exercise, or experiences. If you'd like to share something, please post using **#30DaysNow** or use the exercise's unique hashtag.)

Notes for Day 9

(Use this page to write down thoughts, reminders, ideas, prayers, mantras, revelations, lessons, modifications to the exercise, or experiences. If you'd like to share something, please post using **#30DaysNow** or use the exercise's unique hashtag.)

Notes for Day 10

(Use this page to write down thoughts, reminders, ideas, prayers, mantras, revelations, lessons, modifications to the exercise, or experiences. If you'd like to share something, please post using **#30DaysNow** or use the exercise's unique hashtag.)

Notes for Day 11

(Use this page to write down thoughts, reminders, ideas, prayers, mantras, revelations, lessons, modifications to the exercise, or experiences. If you'd like to share something, please post using **#30DaysNow** or use the exercise's unique hashtag.)

Notes for Day 12

(Use this page to write down thoughts, reminders, ideas, prayers, mantras, revelations, lessons, modifications to the exercise, or experiences. If you'd like to share something, please post using **#30DaysNow** or use the exercise's unique hashtag.)

Notes for Day 13

(Use this page to write down thoughts, reminders, ideas, prayers, mantras, revelations, lessons, modifications to the exercise, or experiences. If you'd like to share something, please post using **#30DaysNow** or use the exercise's unique hashtag.)

Notes for Day 14

(Use this page to write down thoughts, reminders, ideas, prayers, mantras, revelations, lessons, modifications to the exercise, or experiences. If you'd like to share something, please post using **#30DaysNow** or use the exercise's unique hashtag.)

Notes for Day 15

(Use this page to write down thoughts, reminders, ideas, prayers, mantras, revelations, lessons, modifications to the exercise, or experiences. If you'd like to share something, please post using **#30DaysNow** or use the exercise's unique hashtag.)

Notes for Day 16

(Use this page to write down thoughts, reminders, ideas, prayers, mantras, revelations, lessons, modifications to the exercise, or experiences. If you'd like to share something, please post using **#30DaysNow** or use the exercise's unique hashtag.)

Notes for Day 17

Notes for Day 18

(Use this page to write down thoughts, reminders, ideas, prayers, mantras, revelations, lessons, modifications to the exercise, or experiences. If you'd like to share something, please post using **#30DaysNow** or use the exercise's unique hashtag.)

Notes for Day 19

(Use this page to write down thoughts, reminders, ideas, prayers, mantras, revelations, lessons, modifications to the exercise, or experiences. If you'd like to share something, please post using **#30DaysNow** or use the exercise's unique hashtag.)

Notes for Day 20

(Use this page to write down thoughts, reminders, ideas, prayers, mantras, revelations, lessons, modifications to the exercise, or experiences. If you'd like to share something, please post using **#30DaysNow** or use the exercise's unique hashtag.)

Notes for Day 21

(Use this page to write down thoughts, reminders, ideas, prayers, mantras, revelations, lessons, modifications to the exercise, or experiences. If you'd like to share something, please post using **#30DaysNow** or use the exercise's unique hashtag.)

Notes for Day 22

(Use this page to write down thoughts, reminders, ideas, prayers, mantras, revelations, lessons, modifications to the exercise, or experiences. If you'd like to share something, please post using **#30DaysNow** or use the exercise's unique hashtag.)

Notes for Day 23

(Use this page to write down thoughts, reminders, ideas, prayers, mantras, revelations, lessons, modifications to the exercise, or experiences. If you'd like to share something, please post using **#30DaysNow** or use the exercise's unique hashtag.)

Notes for Day 24

(Use this page to write down thoughts, reminders, ideas, prayers, mantras, revelations, lessons, modifications to the exercise, or experiences. If you'd like to share something, please post using **#30DaysNow** or use the exercise's unique hashtag.)

Notes for Day 25

(Use this page to write down thoughts, reminders, ideas, prayers, mantras, revelations, lessons, modifications to the exercise, or experiences. If you'd like to share something, please post using **#30DaysNow** or use the exercise's unique hashtag.)

Notes for Day 26

(Use this page to write down thoughts, reminders, ideas, prayers, mantras, revelations, lessons, modifications to the exercise, or experiences. If you'd like to share online, please post using **#30DaysNow** or use the exercise's unique hashtag.)

Notes for Day 27

(Use this page to write down thoughts, reminders, ideas, prayers, mantras, revelations, lessons, modifications to the exercise, or experiences. If you'd like to share something, please post using **#30DaysNow** or use the exercise's unique hashtag.)

Notes for Day 28

(Use this page to write down thoughts, reminders, ideas, prayers, mantras, revelations, lessons, modifications to the exercise, or experiences. If you'd like to share something, please post using **#30DaysNow** or use the exercise's unique hashtag.)

Notes for Day 29

(Use this page to write down thoughts, reminders, ideas, prayers, mantras, revelations, lessons, modifications to the exercise, or experiences. If you'd like to share something, please post using **#30DaysNow** or use the exercise's unique hashtag.)

Notes for Day 30

(Use this page to write down thoughts, reminders, ideas, prayers, mantras, revelations, lessons, modifications to the exercise, or experiences. If you'd like to share something, please post using **#30DaysNow** or use the exercise's unique hashtag.)

To be mindful is to experience life in the present moment...it's the only moment we have.

Don't forget to leave an online review.

Thank you!

www.ingramcontent.com/pod-product-compliance
Lightning Source LLC
Chambersburg PA
CBHW031247280526
45784CB00004B/1759